Six Days until the Wedding

The Six Day Naturally Beautiful

Regime for That Special Day

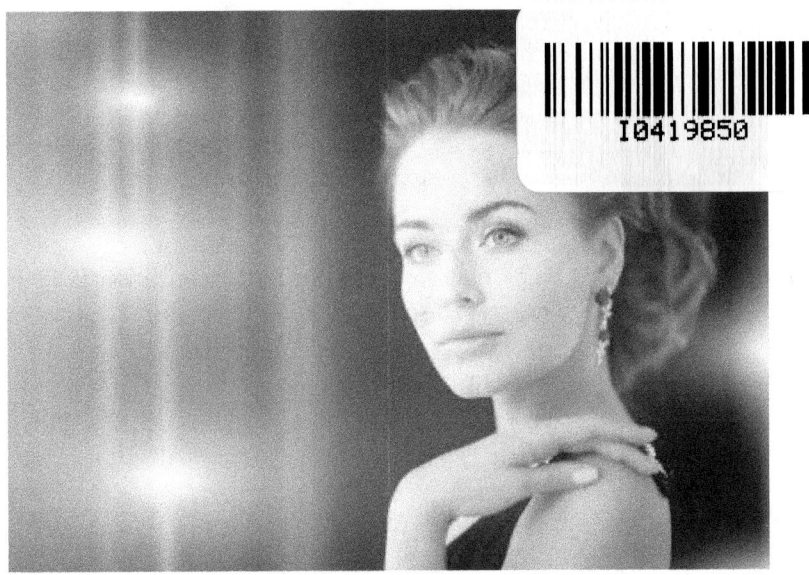

Natural Health Series

Dueep Jyot Singh
Mendon Cottage Books

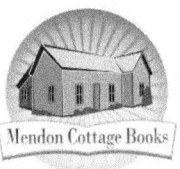

JD-Biz Publishing

Download Free Books!

http://MendonCottageBooks.com

Check out some of the other Health Learning Series books at Amazon.com

Download Free Books!

http://MendonCottageBooks.com

Table of Contents

Introduction

Man is a social being and that is the reason why his life is going to be filled up with social occasions celebrating good times with other like-minded social beings. So naturally if you are fortunate enough to have a full social life with parties, celebrations, and family get-togethers throughout the year, you would want to look just that bit extra scintillating and fascinating, would you not?

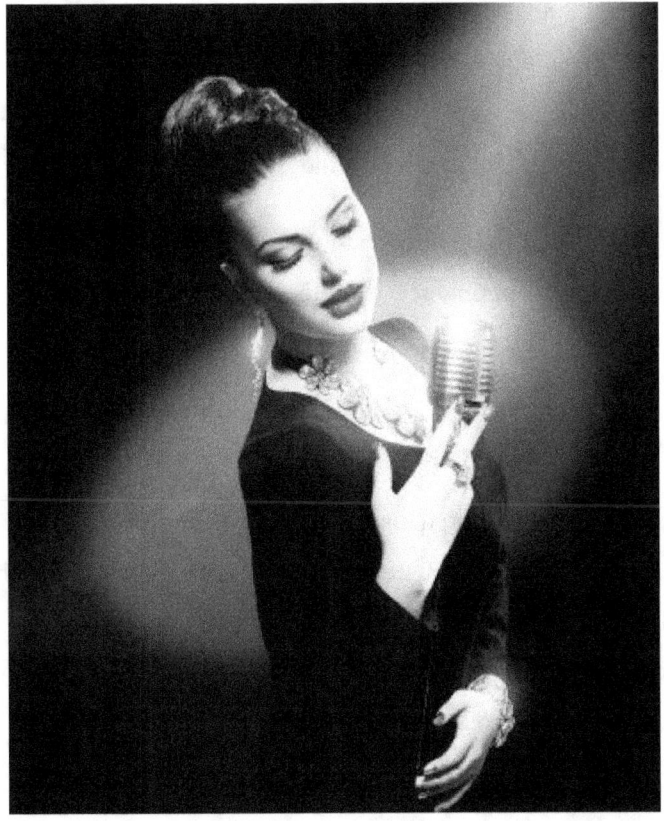

Now she knows how to look good all the time. So can you!

Yes, it is said that beauty is in the eyes of the beholder, but do you know that some of the most "beautiful" women in history were plain looking. But their vivid personality made them really fascinating, and that is why people forgot that they did not have perfect classical Grecian features and the immediate allure of a Venus – Aphrodite. Nevertheless, when you get 1 months prior notice with an unspoken hint of "make sure that you Be There with bells on" and also "here is hoping that the gift that you bring will be substantial," you know that you will need to be looking your best. And if you happen to be the bride, that means that you are going to be the cynosure of all eyes. That puts on that extra burden of you outshining all the other lovelies who have spent the whole month leisurely getting ready for just this occasion, while you rushed around getting things ready for the wedding.

Anyway, this invitation is quite enough for all the women recipients to immediately make an appointment with their favorite beauty parlors, or start to plaster and paste their faces with chemical cosmetics in the hope that they will look exquisitely beautiful on the wedding day and also be the envy of all the other women around them.

It is not necessary to spend so many dollars upon expensive chemical cosmetics when the ingredients are available in right there in your kitchen or easily available in your favorite store.It takes just 6 days for you to know that you are looking your best, that your complexion is glowing and clean and that you are feeling good.

So this six-day regime is going to tone you up from top to toe, and all you have to do is sit back and smiled graciously at the appreciative looks and comments on the day.

Day 6

Remember that a month before the wedding, grooming and care of skin should start if one has been ignoring it earlier. If you have been moving around in the sun, getting things together, and drinking more water and eating healthier foods, including melons and salads, your skin looks radiant. However the problem is that due to sweat and pollution, you may find your skin getting prone to rashes and blemishes and turning it plain dull.

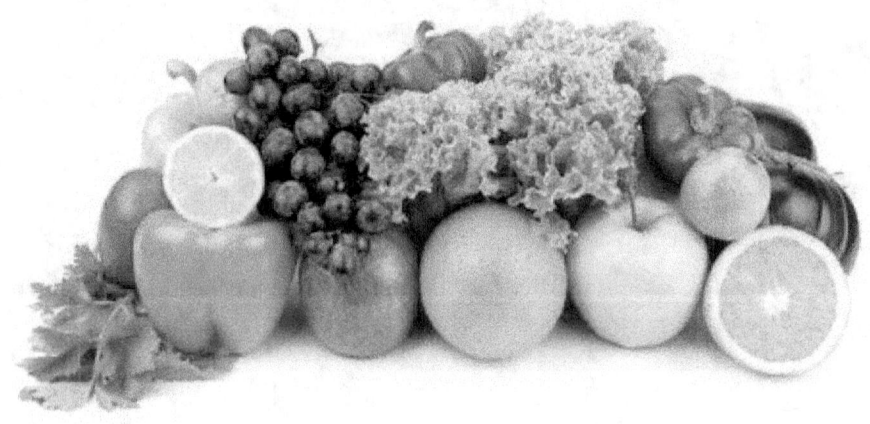

More fruit and more greens keep you healthy and lovely.

So before I start on the six-day regime to wedding day, here are some tips which you are going to do, from the moment you get the ring on your finger and start preparing for the grand occasion. Drink a lot of water and eat healthy food. Stop eating meat. Add more fruit and vegetables to your food. In fact, in the East, soon to be brides are given a diet of fruit and vegetables, so that their skin glows and there is no ammonia smell, which is the side effect of too much meat diet coming out from their body. Also, if you find yourself sweating a lot and especially if you keep on wiping it with dirty hands, increase your fresh fruit juice intake. That is going to keep your body well hydrated. It is also going to keep your skin fresh looking and glowing. If you have to go out in the sun, do it for a short time. To combat the exposure on the harm done to your skin, make a pack as follows –

Combating sun exposure

1 tablespoon coarsely ground sugar

1 tablespoon oatmeal or Fullers Earth.

2 tablespoons yogurt.

Some drops of coconut oil, if your skin is dry.

Mix all these ingredients and rub the mixture on your skin, in gentle and short movements to avoid any rash. This will make your skin glow. This mask is going to dry in 20 minutes, and then you need to remove it by dipping your fingertips in warm water and rubbing off the mixture. Do not rub off any facemask applied on your face, too hard. That is going to exfoliate your skin harshly and leave it raw. You may find yourself with a red red face on the day, instead of the peaches and cream complexion of which you were dreaming.

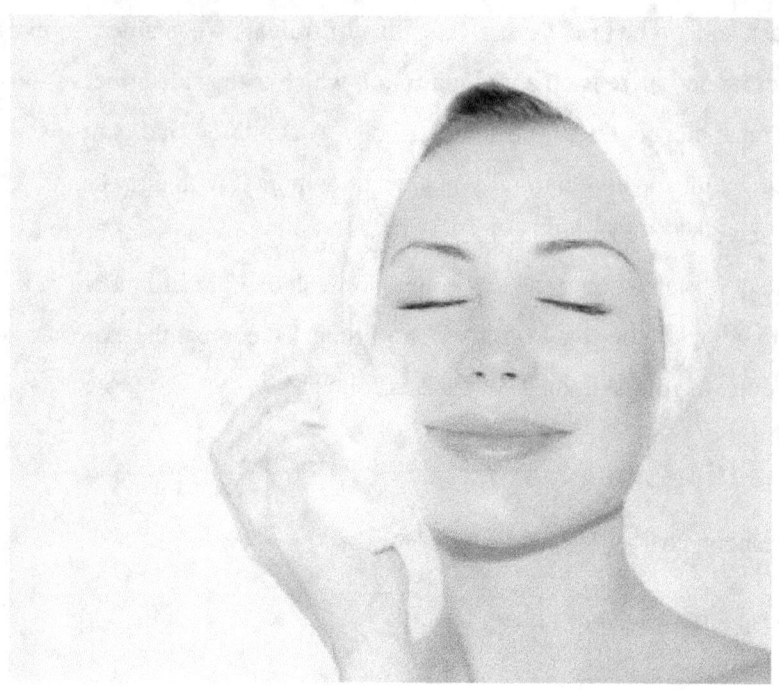

Also, you need to get rid of that winter tan. Although those days spent roasting yourself in the beautiful winter sun is not good for your complexion at all.

Getting rid of winter tan

Take a walnut from your food store of dry nuts and seeds. Powder it well. Put in a little almond oil for moisturizing. Add one teaspoonful of milk and a little rose water and make a paste. Spread it all over your tan skin. Wash it off with warm water after it is dry. Daily application of this mixture will lighten your skin by 3 tones without any recourse to costly and expensive chemical-based skin lightening creams.

For people who want to know what rosewater is – you normally get this rosewater abroad, in expensive bottles, but I am going to show you how you can make your own rosewater.

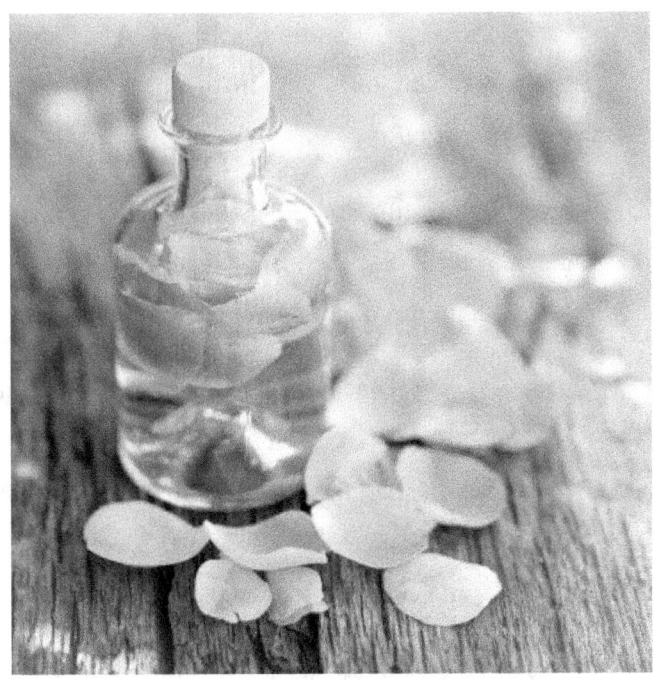

How to make Rose water (Gulab Jal)

Rosewater is normally available in markets at exorbitant prices, but in India, anybody with access to the red rose - Rosa Damascena, - used in India and Iran or Rosa Centifolia which is used in Bulgaria, and Germany-and a little bit of time enjoys making Rosewater at home. This Rosewater is used in cosmetics, as well as in cookery to impart the flavor of the Rose to your meal or to your skin.

Ingredients needed-

1 Cup Rose petals - 12 to 14 flowers.

2 cups water

Lots of ice.

A huge cooking pan - pan number one - with lid in which another pan - pan number two - can be placed comfortably.

Rosewater is just a matter of distillation. Put a wire stand in pan number one, on which you are going to stand the other pan number two. The condensed Rosewater is going to fall into pan number two.

Place the petals at the bottom of the pan number one. Now, cover the petals with water. Place pan number two on the wire stand. Now take the lid and place it upside down on pan number one, thus effectively covering the Rose petals, pan number two and the water. The Rose water is going to condense when you place the blocks and chunks of ice on the inverted lid.

You are going to have a cupful of precious distilled Rosewater, after 25 minutes of slow steaming of the Rose petals.

Precautions - remember to have enough of water to cover the Rose petals. Also, it should not be of such a large quantity, that it displaces the wire stand.

This cooled water is now pure Rosewater. Place it in a sterilized glass bottle. Use it to your heart's content. You may see a little bit of oil swimming over the surface of the water. This is Rose oil, and is even more precious. So if you used lots of petals in a larger pan, you may find even more Rose oil.

This method is for all those people who use a pressure cooker while cooking food. In fact, it is a common way to cook food in Asian kitchens, instead of using the microwave.

You would need water, petals, a pressure cooker and a long thin pipe which it does not melt, when subjected to heat.

Put the water and the petals in the pressure cooker and cover it. Now cover the thin pipe with wet cloth in order to keep it cool. Attach this pipe on the lid of the pressure cooker where you normally attach the weight. Allow the petals to cook slowly, they seem to build up, go through the cooled pipe and collect in a utensil. I tried this way too, but I find the ice on the lid one easier!

Honey lotion

Also, you can use a solution of honey, vinegar, milk and Rosewater mixing one teaspoonful of each as an effective lotion.

Preventing and curing pimples

Can you get mustard seeds anywhere near? The color of the tiny round seeds ranges from yellow to black. They are supposed to be the best Eastern way in which you can cure pimples. In fact, teenagers are recommended by their oldsters in the East to make a paste of mustard seeds soaked in milk for half an hour and then apply this paste on pimples. They can now rest assured that this method will never allow a pimple to raise its ugly head upon their faces.

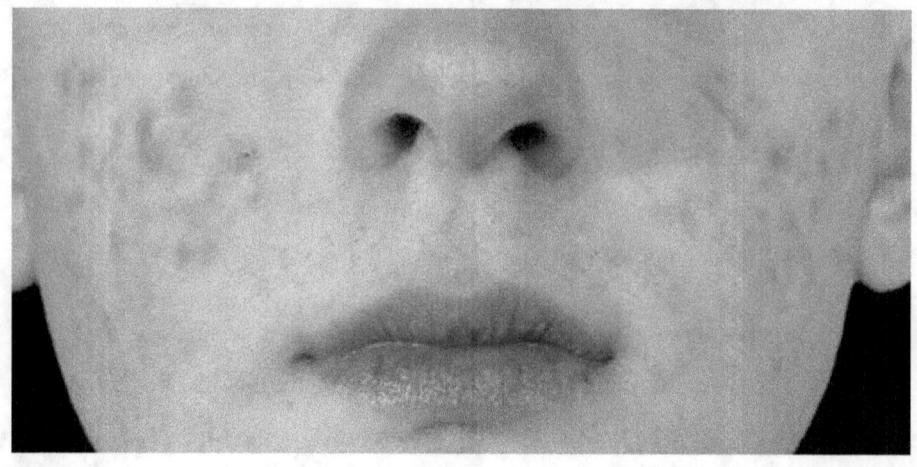

Getting rid of pimples scars

If you have somehow got pimple scars on your face, and you see that it is going to detract from your overall good looks, well, you need to start getting rid of those pimple scars, 3 months before the wedding. Do not try out any chemical process, because that may burn and harm your skin. Instead, start making a paste of turmeric and honey and Rosewater. Apply this paste upon the affected area. If you apply it overnight, make sure that the paste is dry before you go to sleep.

The idea is to heal the skin, while lessening the scars. The next morning, remove this paste with warm water. This is going to exfoliate your skin and encourage fresh skin growth. But if you do not want to keep it overnight, because you are afraid that the turmeric is going to stain the bedclothes, you can apply during the evening and remove it after 30 minutes. Do this regularly until you find your skin glowing naturally and you with a scar free or lightened scars complexion.

Unfortunately, this scar remedy is not going to work if you are deeply scarred, or the scar hurt or injury has gone beyond the upper epidermal layer deep into the lowest epidermis. You would want to talk to a cosmetologist in this case. However, I would suggest that you use makeup to cover these cars, because the cosmetologist may ask you to go in for an expensive chemical-based remedy. How do you know it is going to work successfully? All that money spent with no apparent and visible result.

Firstly, never use any chemical creams, either for cleansing or for moisturizing, however much they are endorsed by your favorite film stars on TV. Many of these films stars do not use those creams themselves, because they know that they are all substance and no promise. Use only creams made from natural recipes for a clean and clear complexion.

Get rid of pimples

You can get rid of pimples, by washing your face with a mild natural soap. Then take a tablespoonful of ordinary sugar and slowly and gently massage it into the skin until the sugar is melted. This drives up all the pimples effectively. If they are quite severe, repeat the treatment for 4 days. Otherwise treatment every alternate day is effective enough.

You are going to learn how to make natural soaps which are good for your skin.

Natural soap

Natural soaps with different essential oils.

Buy a natural soap base at any craft shop. You can normally get glycerin-based melt and pour soap bases with Aloe Vera and honey. As we are just making our own personalized soaps, ¼ pounds of soap base is going to be enough for the first experiment. My friend makes these soaps in earthenware molds, where she just has to break the solidified melted soap and there she is, she has perfect soaps, in shapes, she likes. You can get soap molds in different sizes. They are made of plastic. Choose the soap mold size you want.

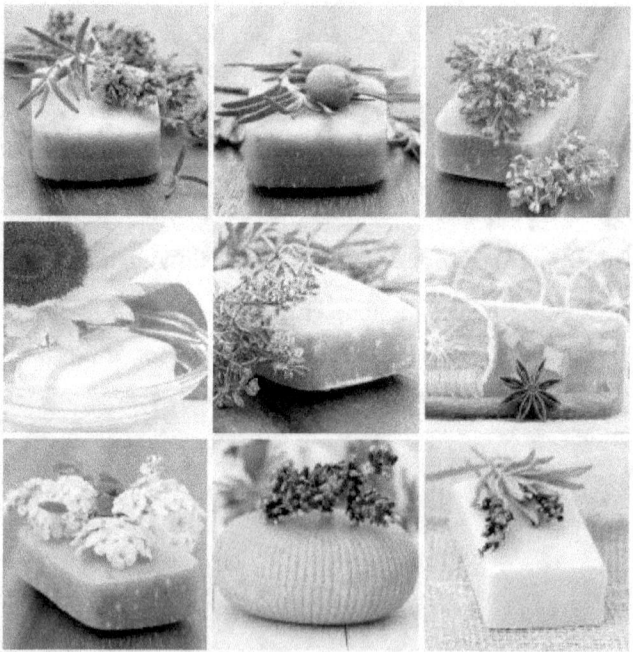

Soap bases are normally without any fragrance. You may like to add your favorite essential oil and coloring. I just put in one – two drops of food coloring to the molten soap base. I melt the base in a pan, placed in another pan full of hot water. This is going to melt the soap, so that it can be poured out into the molds easily. If you want fragrant soap, choose your favorite essential oil, and keep adding 3 – 5 drops of rose oil, lavender oil, or any other oil of your choice, drop by drop, till you reach the required standard of fragrance desired.

Glycerin soaps are best to make natural soaps. Castile soaps have also been made by hand for thousands of years. But as they have lye in it, I am not going to give you the method to make this soap. Do you know that Castile soap was so precious in medieval times that only royalty and aristocrats could afford to buy it. That is why the idea of water and baths being harmful got into the mind of the medieval average man. That is because he was using lye-based homemade soaps upon his skin. The skin got burned, and he decided that the culprit was water, which was the reason why his skin got burned. Cause and effect, no bathing at all, because it burned the skin.

Now that you know how to combat pimples, it is time to moisturize your face.

Prepare a lotion to use after a bath. This **moisturizing lotion** is a lotion which you are going to make a part of your beauty regime, forever, even after your wedding day is long gone.

This is my own personal moisturizing, sunburn – preventing and aging preventing recipe, which was told to me by one of my colleagues who used to make this up every winter with lots of almond oil. I use wheat germ oil, and that is equally effective. Take 125 mL of rosewater. Warm it up gently on a low flame. Add one teaspoonful of lemon juice, one tablespoonful of vinegar, 3 tablespoonful of honey, 2 tables own full of almond oil, or wheat germ oil and hundred milliliters of glycerin to the Rosewater. Heat this mixture up until it is completely blended. She warmed it up; I would recommend placing it in the sun for about 3 hours in a glass bottle and shaking it periodically so that the goodness of the sun gets into it.

Now you can add up little bit of your favorite perfume. I normally add Jasmine essential oil, or rose essential oil to make it smell delicious. Use just a little bit of this every day on your skin. This lotion is perfect to keep your skin well fed. If you feel it is too oily, wipe the skin after 20 minutes.

Now is the time to take care of all the **wrinkles.** I learned this from a friend in Malaysia. Make a mixture of rice powder mixed with lemon juice and honey. Spread it all over the wrinkles and do not move the muscles of your face for 20 minutes. Remove the dried powder with the help of warm water. After this oil your face normally with coconut oil or milk cream. Then rub an ice cube over the wrinkles on your forehead or on your face. This is appealing in the summer, but in the winters, it is most definitely not appealing. She does this every 2nd day. And she is in her 60s, and I must admit, that she does not have any wrinkles. But then she does not expose her skin to the sun, so very often, and cause it to lose essential moisture or spoil its delicate texture.

Day 5

Face bleaching

You may still have this feeling that there is a bit more need for skin whitening. So from tonight onwards, you are going to apply two teaspoons of milk in which a little salt has been added on your face, hands, and neck. You may keep it on overnight. It is going to absorb into your skin, and bleach it. Another bleaching mask is made up with a mixture of yogurt, oatmeal and powdered almonds. This lessens the sunburn and whitens your skin.

Dark circles

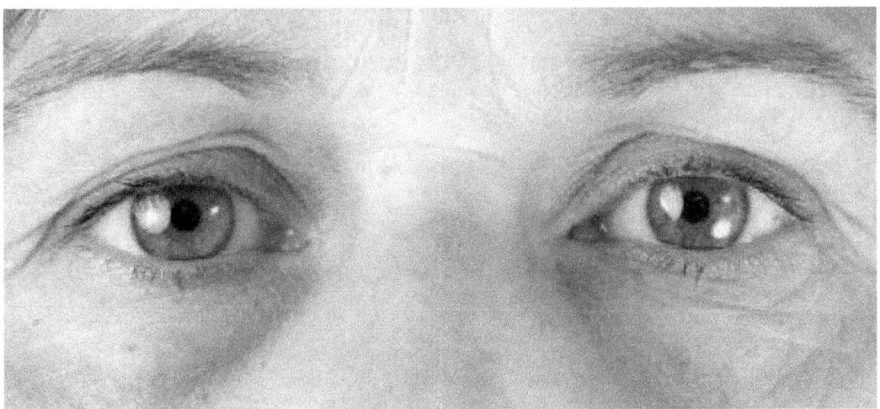

For all those dark circles under your eyes, has it been too many long nights without sleep? We are going to get rid of these dark circles naturally. So start sleeping at 10 o'clock, a month before the day. That is going to reduce the dark circles a lot, unless you are suffering from some ailment which causes them. You need to get fresh air and 8 to 10 hours of regular sleep. You also need to drink 10 – 12 glasses of water every day. If you cannot manage so much water, drink fresh fruit juice. That is even better. Add green leafy vegetables to your diet.

I also love liver, because it has iron in it. Small portions of liver made my way are going to get rid of the iron deficiency in your body.

This recipe is for somebody who wants something delicious and spicy to eat, for lunch or for breakfast before going out on a hard day work. This has nothing to do with being beautiful, but has more to do with getting essential nutrients to stay healthy.

Spiced liver in bread or gurda keema-paranthas

Lamb or mutton mince-keema-1 k.g

Cooked mutton liver- 200 grams, chopped fine.

Onion-2 medium sized

Tomatoes-3 big ones chopped finely.

Green chillies-2 nos

green coriander leaves-1bunch

Garlic-100gms

Ginger-100gms

Salt to taste

chilli powder -2tsp (less for those who are scared of hot spices!)

Turmeric-powder-2tsp

cloves-2 , crushed.

Coriander powder-2tsp

Garam-masala powder-2tsp

Cinnamon powder-1tsp

Cumin-powder-2tsp

Oil or ghee (clarified butter)-2 tbs.

 Heat ghee in the frying pan. Add cumin powder, ground onion, garlic, and ginger into the ghee. Fry on medium flame till golden color. Add all dry ingredients with green chillies and coriander leaves. Now add the keema and the liver to the fried masala. Cover with a lid. Stir keema occasionally to make sure all the masala gets soaked into the meat. It is cooked when it comes away on its own from the sides of the pan. [You can stop this recipe here, if you just wanted a tasty spicy liver-based side dish to eat with rice. But if you want to eat it in bread, carry on reading.]

To make the paranthas, make pastry consistency dough out of flour and let it stay put for half an hour. Then fill the keema into rolls of dough and roll out into 5 inch diameter pastries. The keema has a tendency to escape from the sides, so you can fold the pastries upon each other, by spreading a teaspoon of ghee and then folding the pastry over it into four. Then roll it out again.

Fry on a griddle with ghee applied on the cooked portion. Wash down with creamy milk and curds and with mango pickles.

This cholestrol-laden meal is the centuries old warrior fare of the northern part of the Indian subcontinent and happens to be an addictive breakfast, eaten every morning in many households. This gives the people vim and energy for a day's hard physical work. This is definitely not for those who have a sedentary lifestyle and are just going to go straight to office and hunker down in front of the computer.

A diet of liver and green leafy vegetables is going to remove dark circles, because it is preventing possible anemia. However, if you still want to bleach the dark circles under your eyes, take the juice of one tomato or half a cucumber and add a little turmeric to it. Now make a paste with cornflour, milk and lemon juice. Apply this very carefully under the eyes because this is a very tender and delicate region. Remove it after 20 minutes or after it is dry, with short fingertip movements, with your fingertips dipped in warm water. Do not rub hard. Moisturize this area with the glycerin and rosewater moisturizing lotion. [recipe given above.]

3 – 5 days of application will lessen those dark circles considerably and properly.

So remember, plenty of sleep, and plenty of leafy vegetables will make certain that dark circles will never appear just before that special party or joyous occasion.

Day 4

Tooth bleacher

Today's going to be mouth and tooth care day. You are going to whiten your yellowing teeth, if that has already not been done by the expensive dentist. I would suggest that you start brushing your teeth with a bleaching mixture, 15 days before the wedding. Try a sodium bicarbonate or lemon juice and salt tooth powder. This is the natural whitener. But if you want to make sure that your gums are also trouble free, you will need to use a mixture of mustard oil and salt as a toothpaste with a finger to massage your gums and your teeth. This is the best way to get rid of bad breath, infection inflamed gums and other gum and tooth related diseases.

Bleach your face again with the yogurt, oatmeal and powdered almond mixture, which you did on day 6. That is to lighten your skin tone even more. It is understandable that women want to bleach their skins, but do not go in for artificial bleach at a beauty saloon. It is going to ruin the texture of your skin. It is also going to make your facial hair look golden, while the rest of the hair on your body is still its natural color. I noticed that in one of Madonna's front cover pictures. She had her face and neck bleached. Her facial here was almost invisible. But believe me, the hair on her arms were definitely dark in color. That bleaching had not been done.

Now is also the time to take care of your neck and other neglected portions. These portions like elbows and the knees have to be scrubbed with a loofah. That is to get rid of all the dead cells. Do not use a pumice stone on your heels. Moisturize your face with the moisturizing lotion.

Getting rid of grime on skin

After that, get rid of all the grime on your arms and neck by making up a mixture of one teaspoonful of lemon juice, 1 teaspoon of cucumber juice and milk. Add a pinch of turmeric and dip a piece of cotton wool into it. Clean the dirt and the grime from your neck, elbows and knees with this mixture. You are going to be surprised to know that even when you are fresh out of the shower, after having washed away all that dirt and grime with shower soap, there are still going to be some cells, which still stick on to the epidermis. This lemon juice and milk mixture removes all those stubborn dirt or dead cells.

Skin tightener

Tighten up your skin by making up a mixture of 1 tablespoon of Fuller's earth +1 tablespoon of wheat bran. This mixture is made with 1 tablespoon full of cream. Remove after 30 minutes. Not only is this a good exfoliator, but it tightens up skin wonderfully. After that, you are going to close the open pores by applying a paste of tomato juice. This balances the pH balance of your skin and tomato juice is also an extremely good natural astringent. Now after this is done, you are going to splash your face with cold, cold water, or rub the skin with an ice cube. This gets the tingle back into the skin and closes the pores.

Day 3

Hand care

Today's the day for hand and feet care. Put them into warm water into which one teaspoonful of each – salt and mustard powder – have been added. After this skin has been thoroughly soaked, rub off the dirt, grime and dead cells with a mixture made up of oatmeal, cucumber juice, turmeric and coconut oil. You can use cooking oil to make the solution easily applicable. The moment it dries, rub it off. Now trim your nails, oil them, and then apply your favorite nail polish. This should be a weekly exercise and it should be part of any beauty regimen, irrespective of weddings.

People always admire well-maintained hands, because they are about as much as express and appealing to enhance your personality, as a beautifully made up face is.The time spent on taking care of your hands and can never be thought to be wasted. However, hands and feet only get a fraction of the care we lavish on our faces.

If you think the hand is not expressive, look at the smooth, graceful gestures of a dancer, using her hands to express a variety of emotions. All without speaking. This is sheer poetry and we may have often seen women using their hands so gracefully, even in normal day to day gestures that we feel quite envious.

Being quite human ourselves, we look at our ill cared for, a little treated and rough skinned hands and decide that we shall do something about it – tomorrow. Well, tomorrow is here.

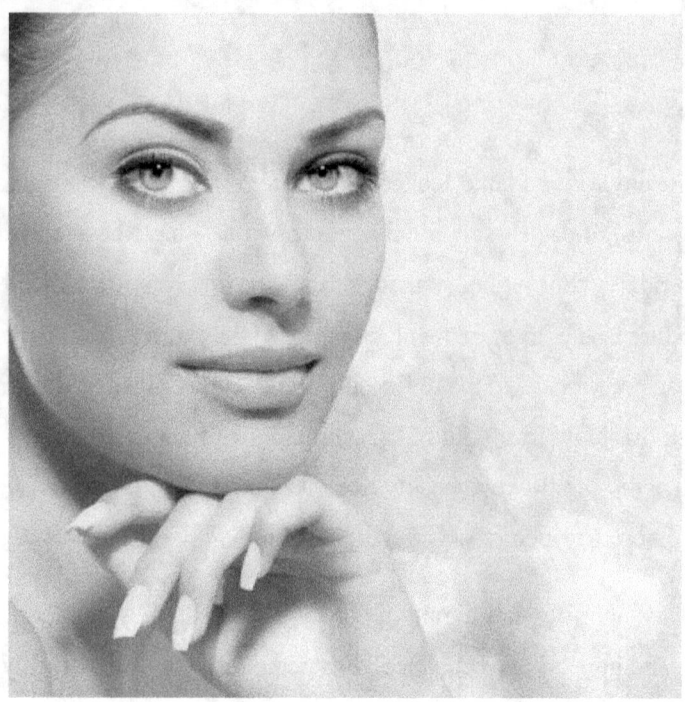

To make your hands look pretty as well as well-kept, start with a manicure. It takes just about to 15 minutes, and once a week is quite enough. In fact, I have found that ordinary water massaged into your hands, while you are watching TV, also works wonders. After all, you are hydrating your hands. Make sure that the massaged movements are toward your heart.

For your manicure, you just need a small bowl of warm soapy water. A small hand towel, a nail file, cotton wool, oil for moisturizing, nail polish remover and your favorite polish. There you are. It is much nicer to polish your fingernails with pink and pearlised shades in the daytime. Nail polish is best applied before you go to bed so that you do not have to worry about badly polished nails in the morning when getting ready for office.

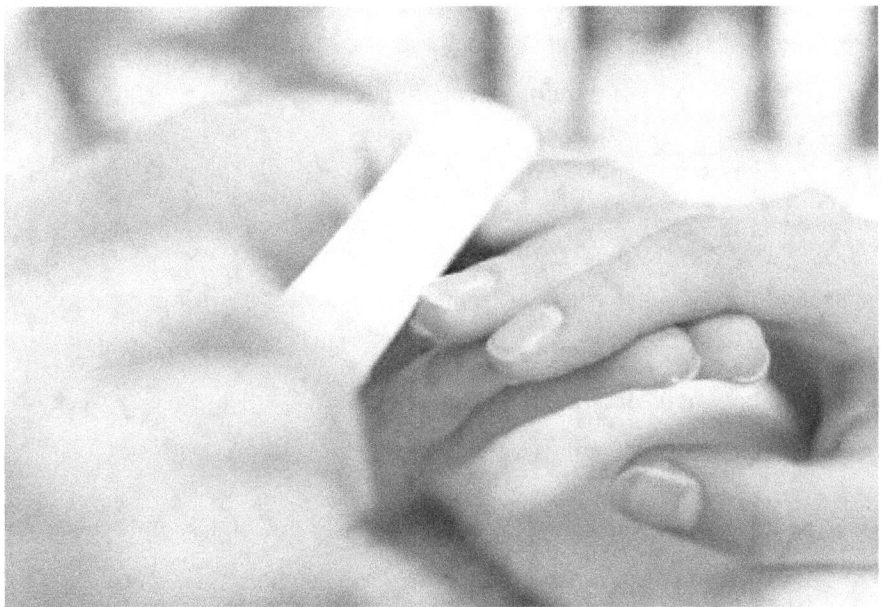

This manicure can be done right at home

Purple violet and other dark shades are a bit to extreme for formal dressing, but if you are getting ready for a party, make sure that the nail polish matches your party dress.

Firstly, remove the older nail polish and then file your nails. Long nails are best suited to people with long slender fingers, and if you have short, study fingers, please make sure that your nails are shaped to an oval, and not more than 1/16 of an inch past your fingertips.

Next soak your hands in the soapy water for 2 minutes. Press back to the cuticles very gently with your towel. They are very delicate and need moisturizing. Do not ever cut your nails so close to the cuticles that they are exposed. They may start to hurt, especially when exposed to rough work.

To remove any soap deposit, wipe your nails again with nail polish remover.

Apply a base coat, beginning with the thumb. Base course are normally transparent nail polishes which are either strengtheners, or just present to stop the chemical products of your nail polish from yellowing your nails. I normally let my nails breathe free without nail polish at least once a week, so that I do not suffer from yellow nails.

After the base coat has been applied, apply the nail polish. Use only two light coats, allowing the 1st to dry completely before you apply the 2nd coat. Finally, when the polishes complete the dry, massage the coconut oil into your hands up to your wrist to moisturize and oil the skin.

Please make it a rule be removed or original nail paint before applying any new nail polish. A manicure once a week keeps your hands feeling good. As it is always preferable to use natural products rather than expensive creams and moisturizers go back to nature and every night, use just a bit of milk cream or milk as a natural moisturizer. a little bit of salt added to it will bleach your hands beautifully..

Keeping your legs beautiful

So alright, not all of us have legs like Marlene Dietrich or Betty Grable. What really means beautiful legs depends on the shape and their length. The one test of beautifully shaped legs is standing with feet together and see if you can hold a coin between your ankles, another between your calves and another between your knees, all at the same time. That is tough!

Beautiful legs normally have a space between ankle and calves and between calves and knees. But do not think that your legs are not beautiful, if you do not have these proportions. Many ladies think that their legs are too fat or too thin, just because they do not pass the space test. Unfortunately, the actual shape of your legs cannot be easily changed. However, with exercise you can improve muscle tone and make them look better.

Lose fat by going on a sensible diet by cutting down on potatoes, rice, and adding up on poultry, fish, eggs and cheese with fresh fruit and vegetables. If you have too thin legs, improve them with exercises. Your legs can look much more shapely with regular exercising and muscle building.

Leg exercises

Put your heels together. Rise on your toes. Sink to the ground. Bending your knees back, straight and then get up slowly. This exercise has to be repeated 3 times, and it is sheer cruelty. But it works.

Walking and bicycling are wonderful exercises for getting shapely legs. In the office , walk up the stairs instead of taking a lift.

Sometimes legs may not be fat, but look heavy. That is because of bad circulation. Would your legs and feet up in case you have the feeling of water retention, drink about 6 glasses of water. This is going to get all the toxic accumulated wastes out.

Smooth legs look more appealing than fuzzy legs. The best natural hair remover is a turmeric paste, applied before a bath. After it has dried, rub off the turmeric paste. And then have your bath. Regular use of this paste is going to remove your hair naturally and discourage hair growth. Turmeric hair remover is also used to discourage hair growth on the face and other parts of your body since ancient times. Moisturize your body after using a turmeric hair remover

The way you walk also has a great effect on your personality. If your walk is like a camel marching straight across the desert with your knees bent, well, march on, dromedary. The legs must be straight and the walk should be from the hips. Your toes must touch the ground first, followed by the heel. Striding ladies looked good only in uniform! The steps must be dainty and the foot must be placed before the other, as if you are stepping on an invisible line on the floor. Of course your head should be up, shoulders back, and back erect and this is going to do wonders for your personality. Do not hold your neck stiff.

Stylish sitting pose

Also, remember that when you are going to be sitting at the party, your style of sitting is going to be either stylish or just plain sloppy. Crossing your legs may look stylish when you are wearing trousers or when you think yourself a tomboy, but they detract from your appeal. Also, sitting with legs spread is good enough for men, but women look crude, if they sit in that fashion.

I got this tip from a model friend, who got it from an old movie star's TV interview somewhere in the 60s. Ordinary legs can look beautiful when you sit with your legs not crossed and parallel to each other with the left foot slightly behind the right ankle. This sitting style looks amazingly good, when you are wearing heels. The legs should be leaning to one side, side-by-side. Hands should be placed in front of you, showing them off and should be used occasionally to emphasize a point in a gracious and graceful gesture.

Do not use your hands over much when you are talking to people. That distracts. I notice Meg Ryan does this a lot. Her hands do more talking than she does, especially when she is trying to say "go, go, go away." The hands start gesturing even before she has said the words and still keep moving even after she has finished saying them. Many of us do this, especially when we are thinking up what to say next. It can get plain scary, especially when the hands are long fingered.

Did anybody see the Oliver Reed starring comedy *Hannibal Brooks*? Michael J Pollard played a dopey escapee POW named Packy with delusions of military grandeur and glory . His acting was hilarious, but one kept getting distracted and wondering whether he was high on something. That was because his well shaped hands with long, bony fingers kept gesticulating and moving all the time. Plain scary and makes one wonder about the state of the speaker's mind.

So now that you know how to keep your hands and legs beautiful, try these tips on day 3. In this way both your hands and your legs shall be focus points, giving you a hands down and a leg up advantage anywhere you go.

Day 2

Removing blackheads

This is the day when we are going to get rid of the blackheads on our nose. Funny, this is one thing that we do not look at, very often. The nose accumulates a lot of grime, and even cleansing may not remove those unsightly blackheads. Make up a mixture of 1 teaspoon of ordinary baking powder with some oatmeal and water. Apply this paste all over the nose and rub off when it is dry. Some women prefer to drop the nose with wheat bran soaked in milk. I find the baking soda less painful.

Body odor

Just take a handful of mint leaves, add a handful of rose petals and add the rind of 2 lemons to it. Boil with 2 cups of water. Leave this solution overnight.

The next day strain and bottle up this natural deoderant. Whenever you take a bath, apply it all over your body and let it dry. Who needs chemical deoderants when you can get a natural body natural sweet smelling solution to prevent body odor.

Hair care

In the 1940s, a company named WH Fitch sold Fitch's saponified coconut oil shampoos, which supposedly cured dandruff. I do not know what they added to that shampoo, but this much I know that shikakai and soap nuts have an ingredient called saponin. So we are going to be making a herbal shampoo, today, which we are going to use on day one.

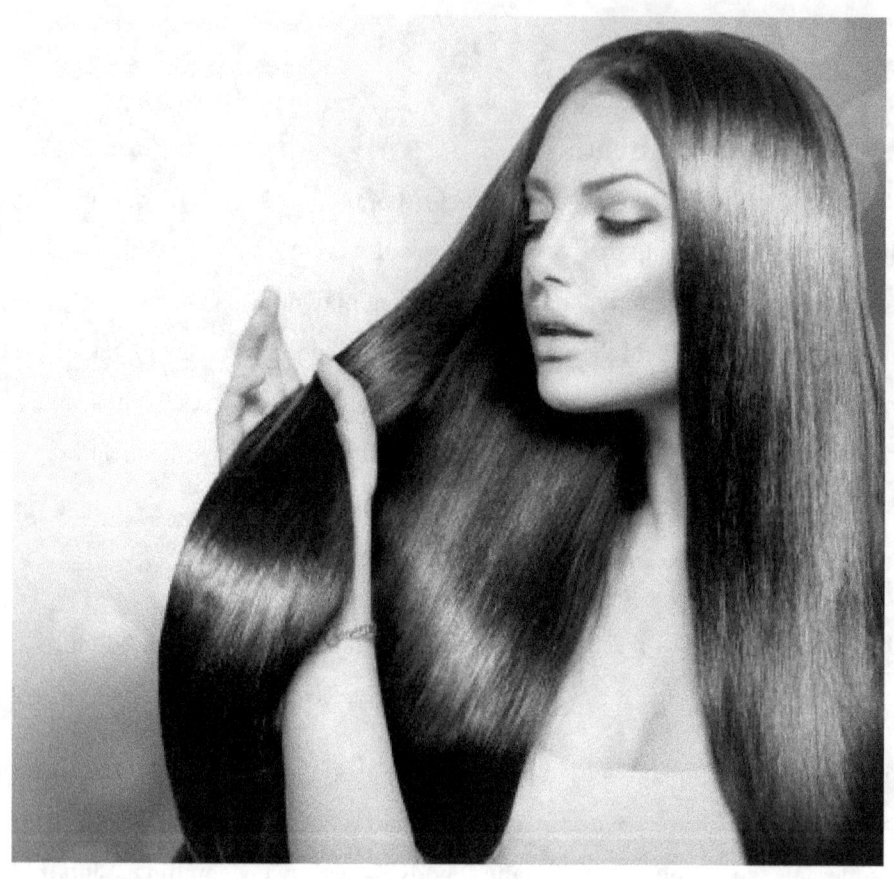

Take two soap nuts,(http://en.wikipedia.org/wiki/Sapindus) two pods of shikakai ,(http://en.wikipedia.org/wiki/Acacia_concinna) 2 tablespoons of dried gooseberry powder and 1 hibiscus flower and powder them together. You may leave them overnight in an iron vessel with 2 cups of water, if you intend to concentrate on hair care on day one.   This herbal shampoo has to be boiled until the 2 cups are reduced to 1 cup. Strain the solution, which is going to be used as a shampoo.

Remember that if you are blonde or do not have dark-colored hair, do not soak this solution in an iron utensil. The soaking in the Iron utensil is to darken the hair and make it jet black, without the use of chemicals based dyes.

Now you are going to do the massaging of your hair so that it is silky smooth tomorrow. Massage your scalp with a bit of warm oil. Coconut oil is best, because it is considered to be a really good nourish her of your scalp. For the oil to get really absorbed so Towel in hot water. Squeeze it and wrap it for 20 minutes around your head. After 20 minutes, you can shampoo your hair with the liquid herbal shampoo and in the last rinse, use the juice of one lemon mixed with ¼ mugs of water. And see people taking a shine to you and your lovely hair.

I normally do this on day one, so that my hair still feels freshly shampooed. That means that I sleep with my hair oiled overnight. You do not need another conditioner, once it has been treated to the coconut power.

Day 1 - The Special Day

Today's the day when you intend to relax, especially when you know that it is going to be hectic in the evening. Stop hurrying about in a harried fashion. Plenty of worry and scurry may just spoil the curry and make you so exhausted that you may not find yourself able to enjoy the party at the appointed hour.

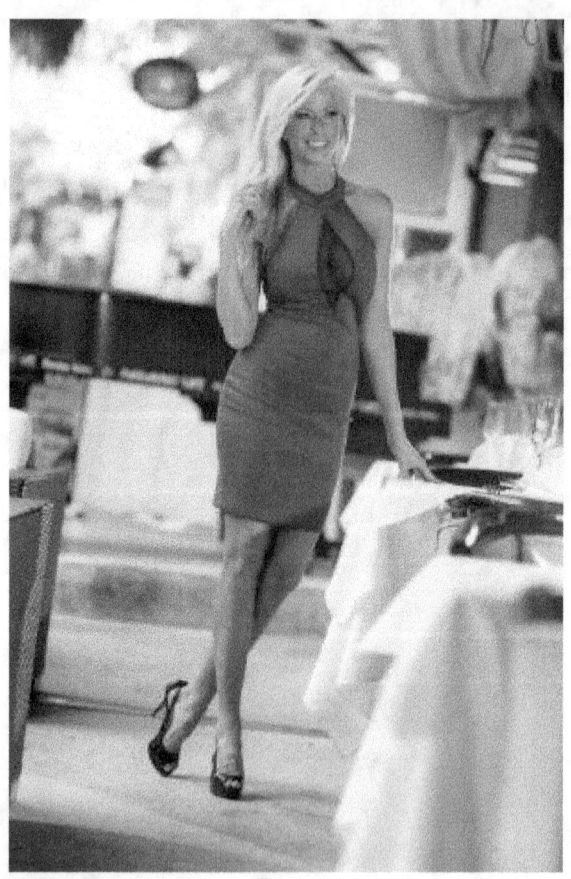

Make sure that your clothes are well pressed and clean. Check for loose buttons. Buttons have a bad tendency of falling off at the last moment. Do not drench yourself with your favorite scent just to show everybody that it has come straight from Paris. Subtlety is style!

About 200 years ago, one of the most famous arbitrators of British fashion George "Beau" Brummel spoke these famous words. "Make sure that your dress is perfect in all ways. And then forget about it."

What he meant was that many times he saw people twitching their dress, fiddling with it, and fussing ever so often to make sure that the folds fell perfectly, or anything else. What is the use of beautiful brooches and discrete safety pins, if not to make you forget about portions of your dress, which are liable to flow loose or slipping off East, when you are going West? This is going to be almost on par to Jayne Mansfield's much-publicized wardrobe malfunctions, which started out as a publicity stunt, but began to lose its novelty when it was repeated on every possible occasion.

So now that you know that you are looking good, it is time to feel good. Lift up your head high and smile.

Remember to pick up a small matching purse with these items in it – money, lipstick, mouth spray [a small airline toothpaste and toothbrush is also handy] small hand mirror, a small comb, tissue, safety pins, handkerchief, pen and paper and even a needle and thread. This list comes from experience.

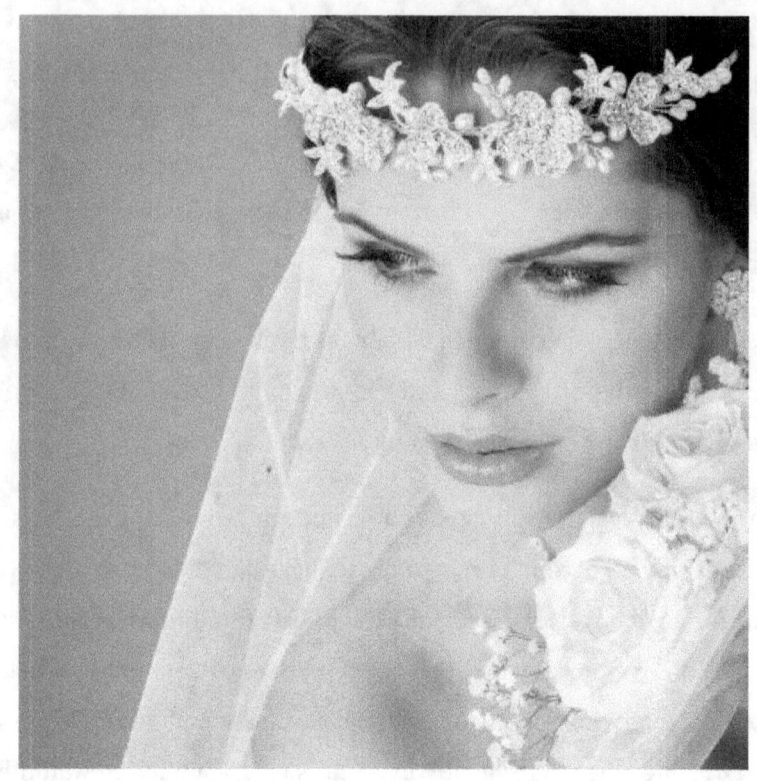

I remember attending the wedding of a relative, well made up with perfect war paint. The moment we reached the venue, we heard that they were going to feed us first before the wedding ceremony took place. So you can understand what happened. Eating and drinking lots of delicious, spicy food , outdoors on a windy day without any lipstick, comb and mouth spray. Had to keep my mouth shut throughout the ceremony, and even afterwards because I knew I would be smelling of spicy delicious lunch dishes. So celebrations are for enjoying, and enjoy your wedding day. Also, remember to switch off your cell phone during the ceremony, because you do not want to spoil the emotional and touching moment of " I do "being disturbed by "Braaa-zeeeel, nananananana…"

Been there, seen or rather heard that! And the embarrassed guest fumbling for his phone and saying excuse me Excuse me, sheepishly as he stumbled out of the wedding venue.

Conclusion

So now, you know all about the beauty, grooming, and personality tips and techniques, which are going to make you the cynosure of all eyes, on a special occasion, try them out right now. Most of these techniques are general, and which you are going to use in your own beauty regime. Others are special techniques, which are normally used by beauticians, but as we are talking about natural based tips, you are going to find them much more economical, time-saving, effective and beneficial to you in the long run.

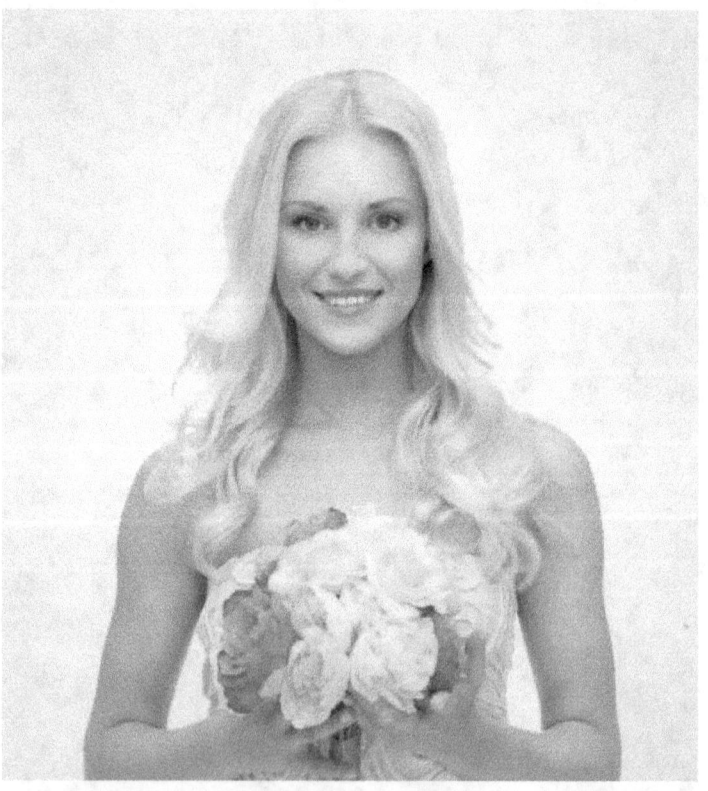

Remember that the elements of feeling beautiful is to respect yourself and think yourself second to none. This is going to give you the assurance that you look your best, especially when you feel your best. a little bit of care in just 6 days are going to make a major drastic change in your life and in your lifestyle. You do not have to restrict this regime to just one special occasion. You can use it every day of your life, Sunday through Saturday.

So enjoy your wedding day and live life Emperor size.

Author Bio

Dueep Jyot Singh is a Management and IT Professional who managed to gather Postgraduate qualifications in Management and English and Degrees in Science, French and Education while pursuing different enjoyable career options like being an hospital administrator, IT,SEO and HRD Database Manager/ trainer, movie scriptwriter, theatre artiste and public speaker, lecturer in French, Marketing and Advertising, ex-Editor of Hearts On Fire (now known as Solctice) Books Missouri USA, advice columnist and cartoonist, publisher and Aviation School trainer, ex- moderator on Medico.in, banker, student councilor ,travelogue writer … among other things! One fine morning, she decided that she had enough of killing herself by Degrees and went back to her first love -- writing. It's more enjoyable! She already has 48 published academic and 14 fiction- in- different- genre books under her belt.

When she is not designing websites or making Graphic design illustrations for clients who want Walt Disney, Norman Rockwell , JJ Grandville or Hed Kandy type illustrations, she is busy browsing in old bookshops for antique books,-she has a mouthwatering collection of priceless First editions and rare books…including R.L. Stevenson, O.Henry, Dornford Yates, Maurice Walsh, C.N.Williamson, and the crown of her collection- Dickens "The Old Curiosity Shop," and so on… Just call her "Renaissance Woman") - collecting herbal remedies, making one of a kind creations in Irish Crochet and Aran knitting, acting like Universal Helping Hand/Agony Aunt, or escaping to her dear mountains for a bit of exploring, collecting herbs and plants , trekking, and rappelling.

Gardening Series on Amazon

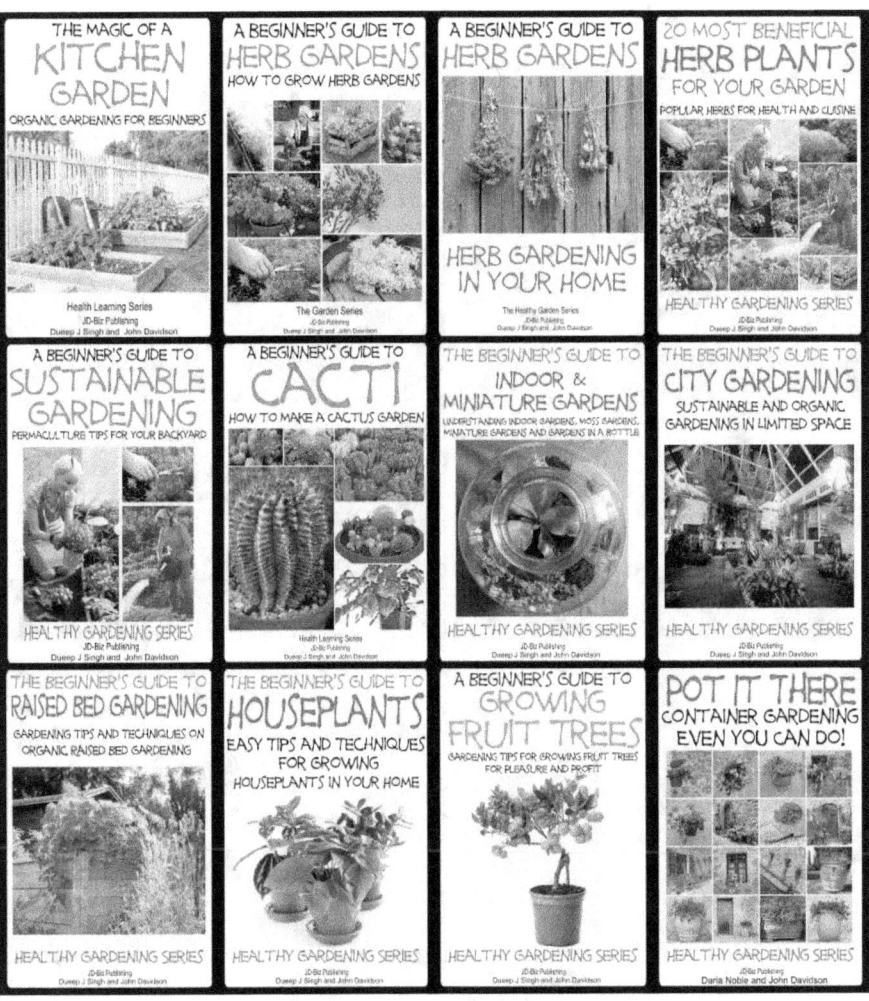

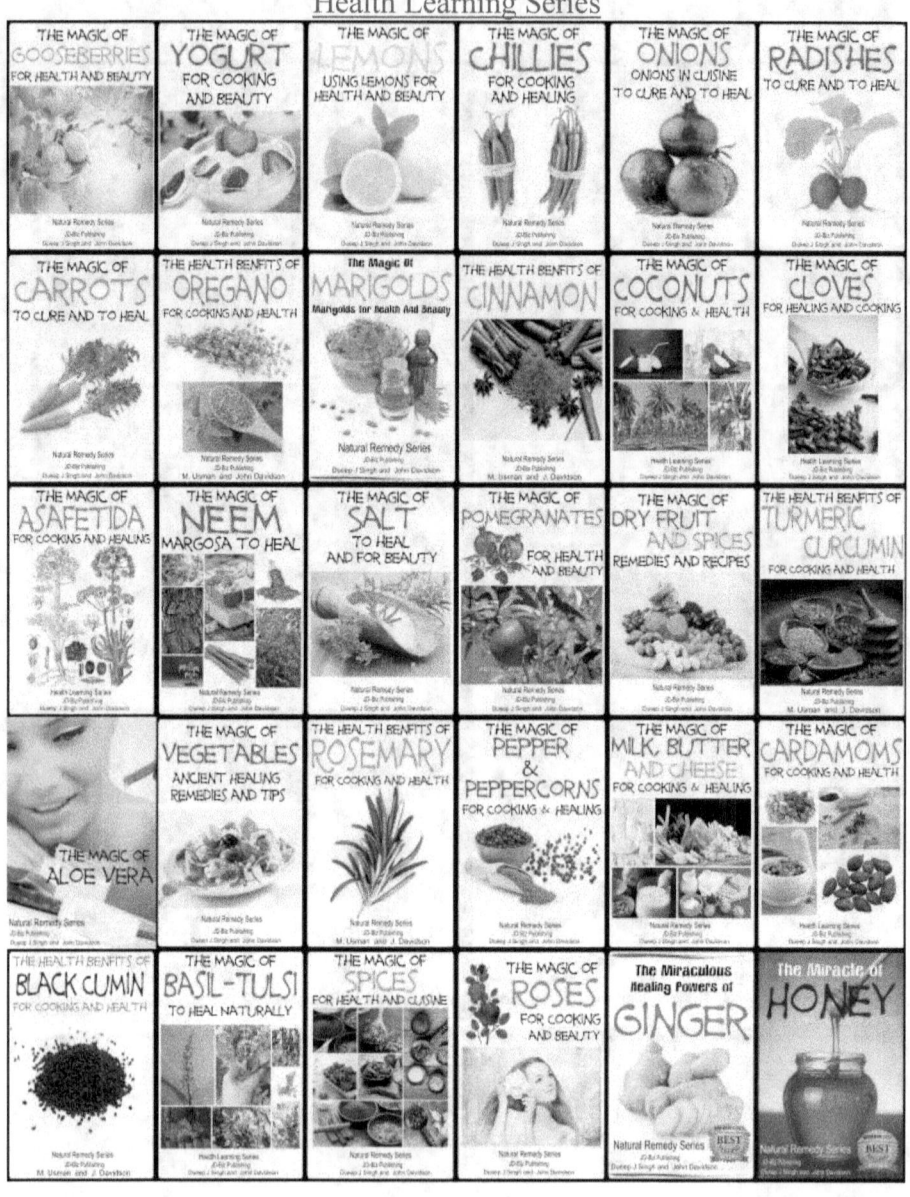

Country Life Books

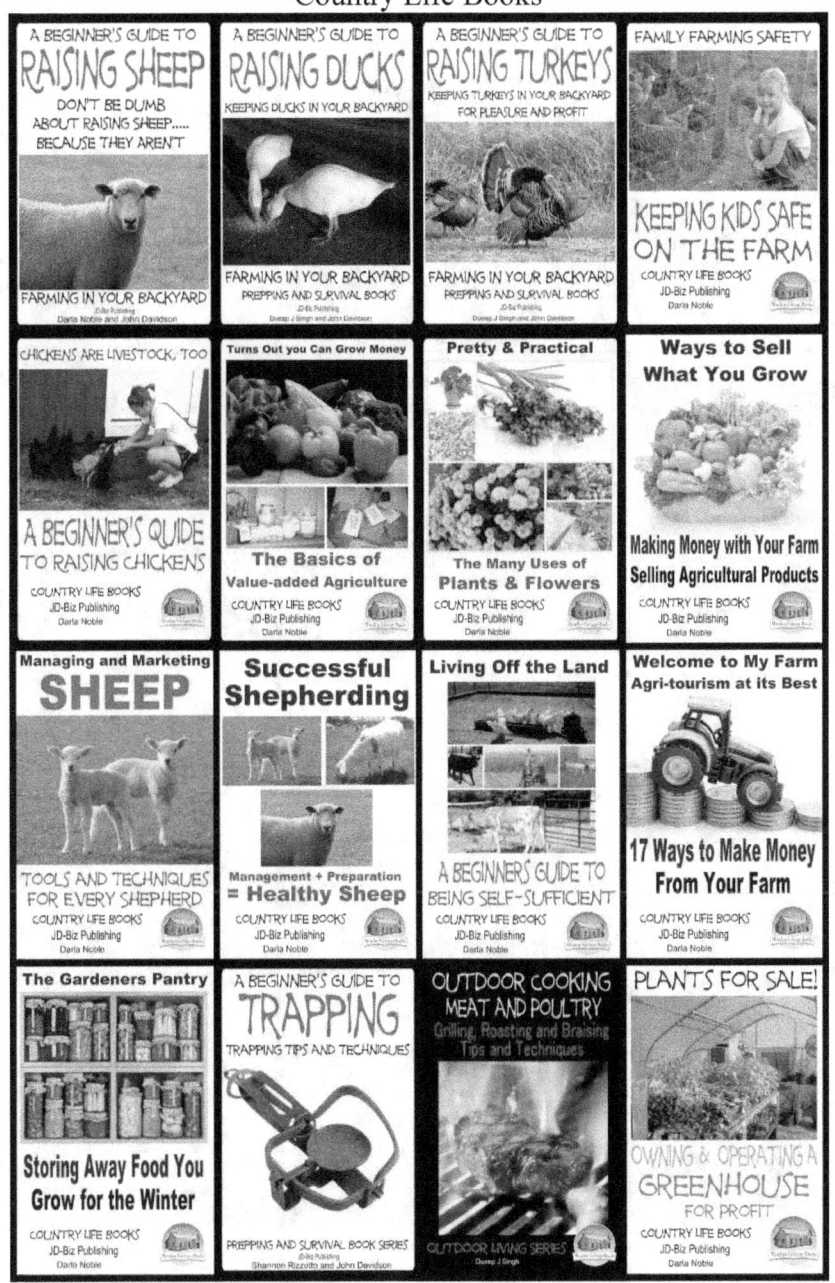

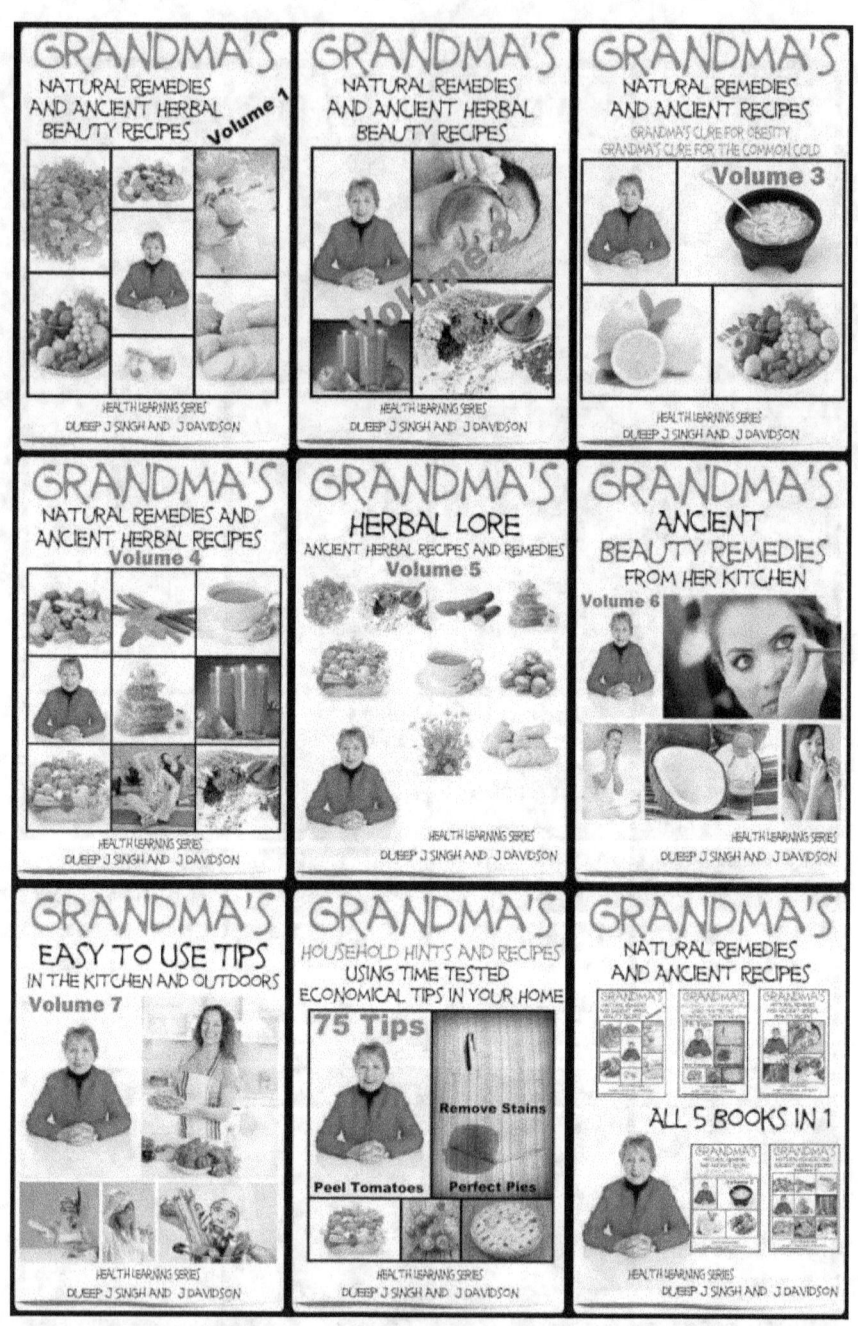

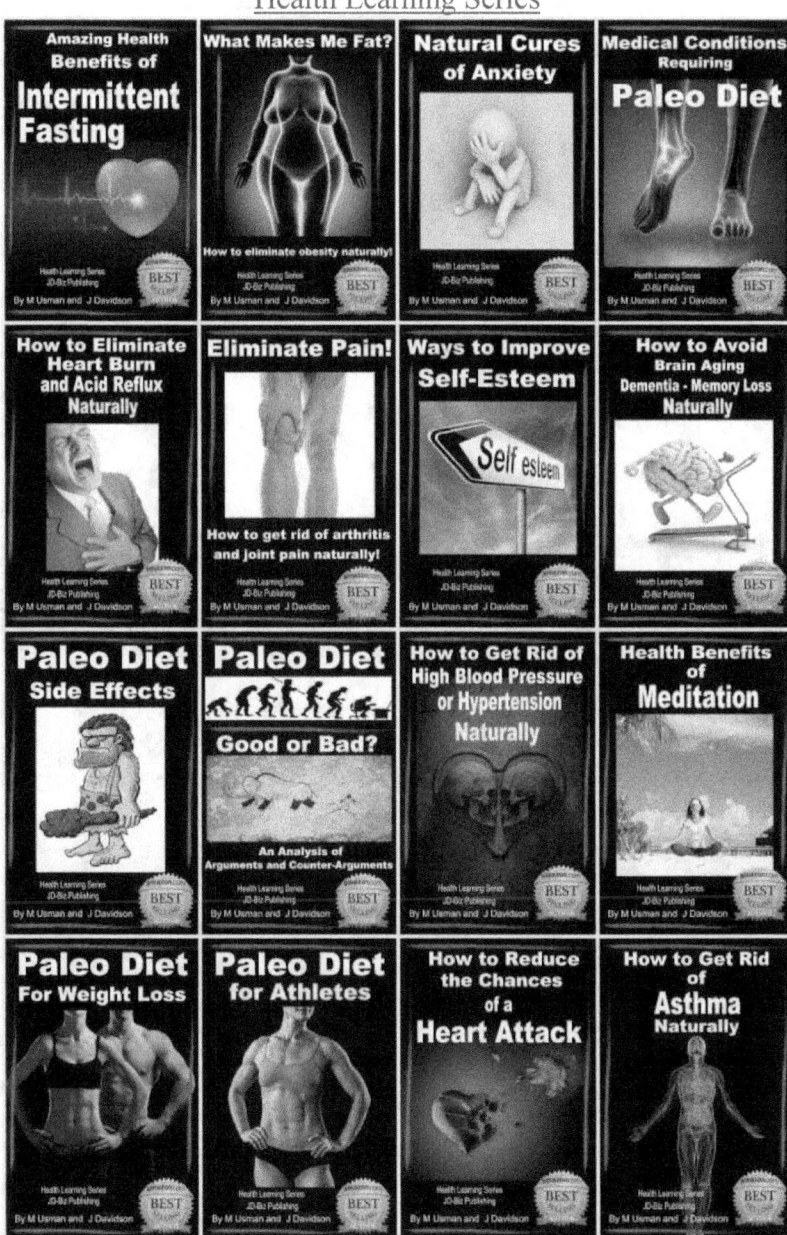

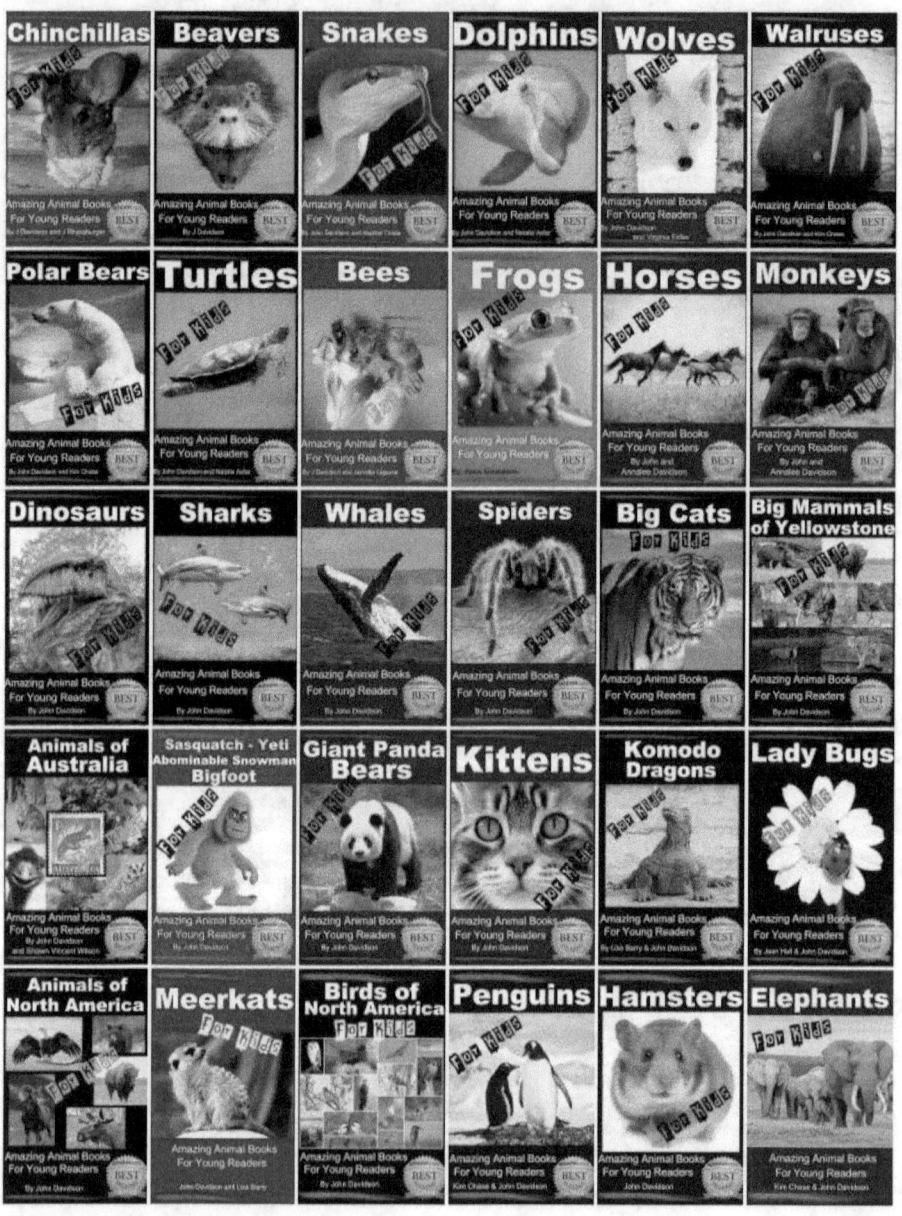

Learn To Draw Series

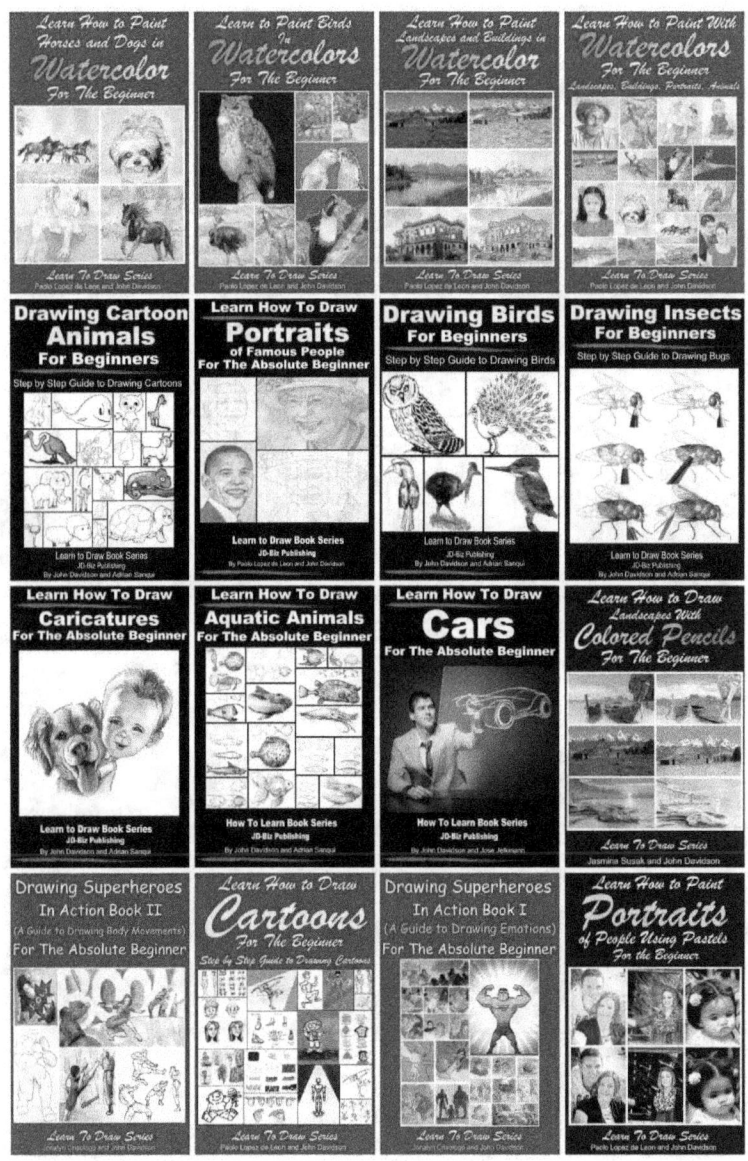

How to Build and Plan Books

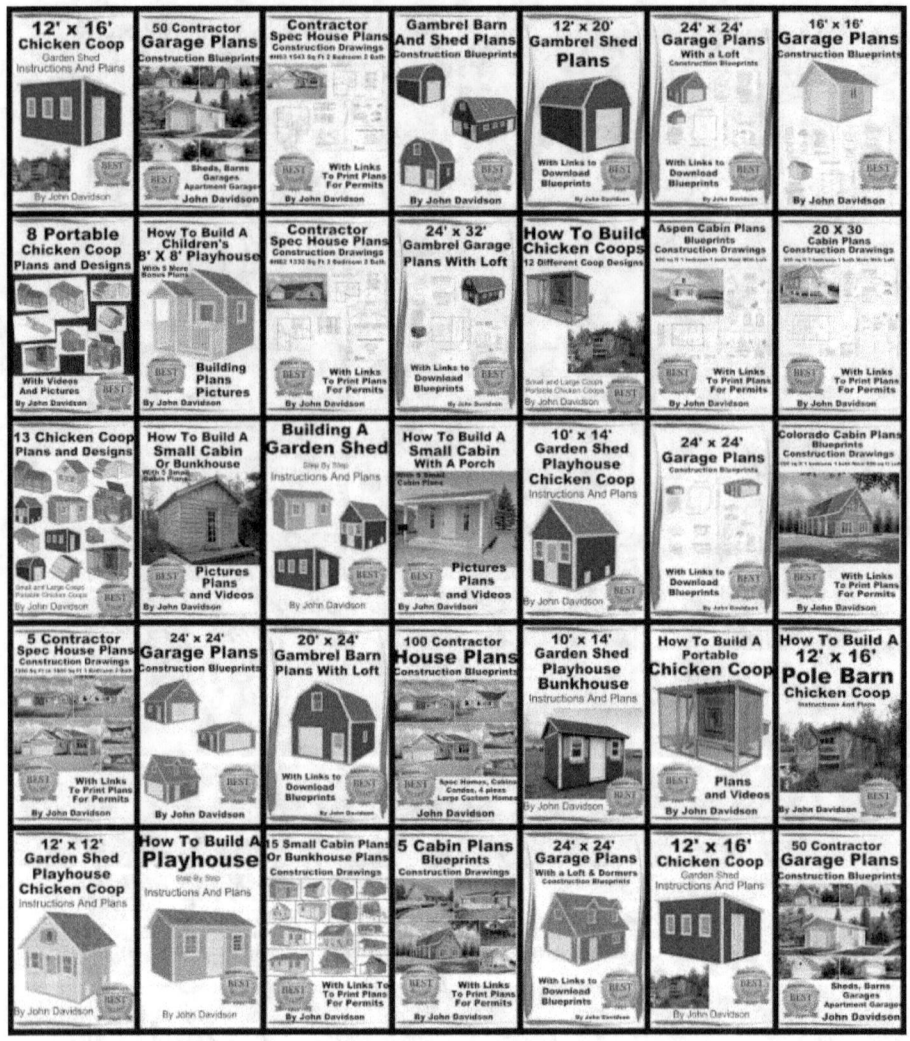

Entrepreneur Book Series

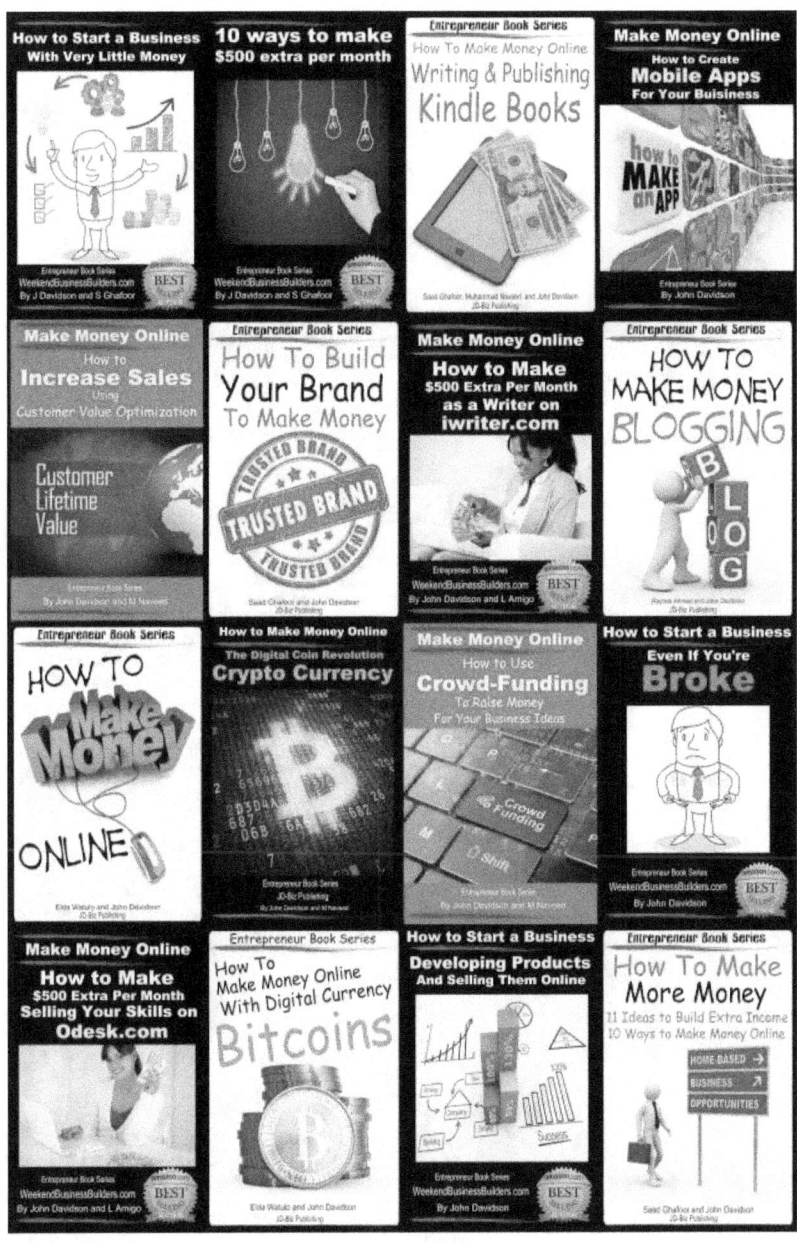

Our books are available at

1. Amazon.com
2. Barnes and Noble
3. Itunes
4. Kobo
5. Smashwords
6. Google Play Books

Download Free Books!

http://MendonCottageBooks.com

Publisher

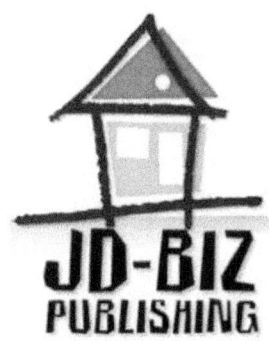

JD-Biz Corp

P O Box 374

Mendon, Utah 84325

http://www.jd-biz.com/

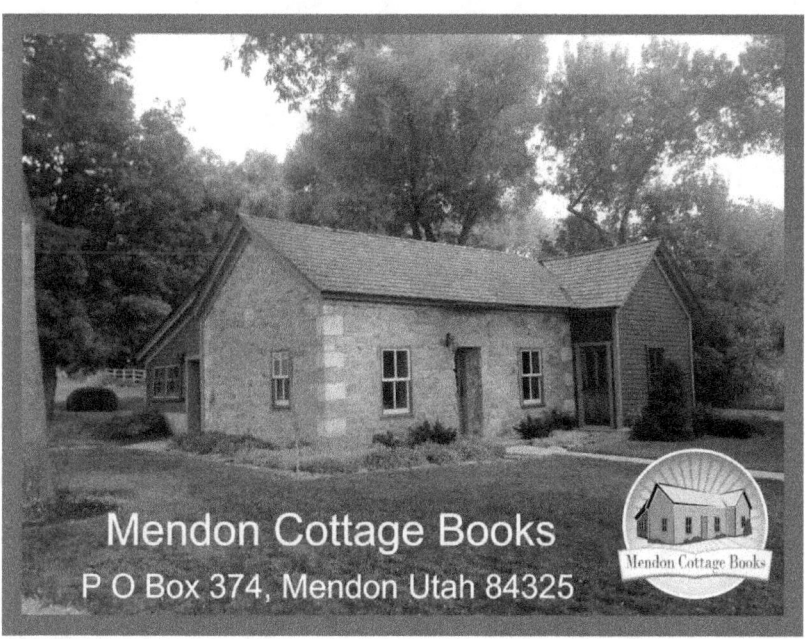

www.ingramcontent.com/pod-product-compliance
Lightning Source LLC
Chambersburg PA
CBHW071132280526
45787CB00003B/1248